ASHLEY LUMPKINS

Healthy Kid Hacks

8 Hacks to Healthy, Happy Kids that Won't Break the Bank

This book was professionally typeset on Reedsy.
Find out more at reedsy.com

Contents

Introduction

For years, I've had friend after friend tell me I should write a book or start a blog to share all my natural tips and tricks that I use on a daily basis to help keep my kiddos healthy, so here we are.

A little back story on my own health journey, I struggled with chronic allergies and multiple sinus infections for most of my adolescence through young adulthood. I was constantly on some sort of an allergy medication and nasal spray prescribed by my pediatrician. Every time I got sick, I was hit with a round of antibiotics. There was no education on how to heal or prevent allergy symptoms and sinus infections naturally, just pharmaceuticals.

In my early twenties, I was determined to discover a better way. Surely there must be an alternative to this vicious cycle?! I popped into a natural wellness store in St Augustine, FL, and received some advice and guidance that changed my life that day. I was taught how to heal my body naturally, and I quickly became passionate about telling others how they could do the same.

Over a decade later, I became a mom for the first time so naturally this mindset and lifestyle approach carried through in how I raised my children. It's been over 6 years of "momming" these precious kids as I write this. It has not always been easy, as honestly, the path we choose is not the most-trodden one. Many of my choices were frowned upon by others. I appeared "over the top" to some family members and friends, but my convictions were too strong to care about their opinions. I had seen the benefits of this lifestyle first hand and I knew I needed to train them up early. Even if they stray from my guidance one day, I will know I did my best to give them a solid foundation.

What to expect from this book

This book does not have any miracle cures and certainly won't fix all your problems as a parent, but I do hope it will be a useful and simple tool to help move you in the direction of creating healthy, happy kids.

I'm not writing this to sell you on any particular product or company, but I will list some of my preferred vendors at the end of the book in case you were wanting some recommendations. There are so many choices out there, it can be overwhelming to figure out where to start.

While I could probably write a few more books to hit all the things, I have chosen 8 "hacks" to focus on for this book. These are some of the most important areas to educate yourself in if you desire to create healthier, happier kiddos, and I'm guessing you do because you're here. Let's jump right in!

1

Hack #1 Change the Environment

I don't know about you but I grew up in a home that used every day, grocery store cleaning and laundry products that were filled with noxious fumes and WARNING labels. I remember the cleaning products were so strong, I could taste them. I'd have to take breaks to get fresh air while cleaning the bathroom as I coughed on the fumes. It was normal to throw some bleach in your laundry load and spray disinfectants and deodorizers everywhere.

Maybe this is still your normal, and that makes me so glad you're here reading, learning and evolving. When we know better, we do better. Now, don't get me wrong, I know it's hard to change. Trying new things can be daunting and even overwhelming. Don't feel like you have to suddenly change everything you do. You can take action towards simple, consistent changes over time.

The fact of the matter is, national brand cleaners that you see every day on shelves across the US, and likely have in your cabinets, are filled with toxic ingredients that are damaging our health. A 20 year long, independent study completed by the American Thoracic Society found that using national brand cleaners as little as once a week is as damaging to our lung capacity as smoking a pack of cigarettes a day for 20 years. Say what?! Yes, that's what I said too! The American Lung Association warns against the use of national brand cleaners, stating the dangerous chemicals, including toxic VOCs, that are released into the air when these products are used leads to chronic respiratory illnesses, allergies, asthma, headaches and more.

Okay, hopefully I've stressed enough why we need to make changes, so let's talk about what we need to do to actually make the shift towards a healthier home environment. This topic can get overly complicated fast, so I'm going to keep it simple and give you a list of things you should absolutely avoid using in your home to get you rolling in the right direction.

The "No" List:

- Chlorine Bleach
- Ammonia
- Abrasives
- Phosphates
- Phthalates
- Triclosan
- Parabens
- Formaldehyde
- Quaternary Disinfectants

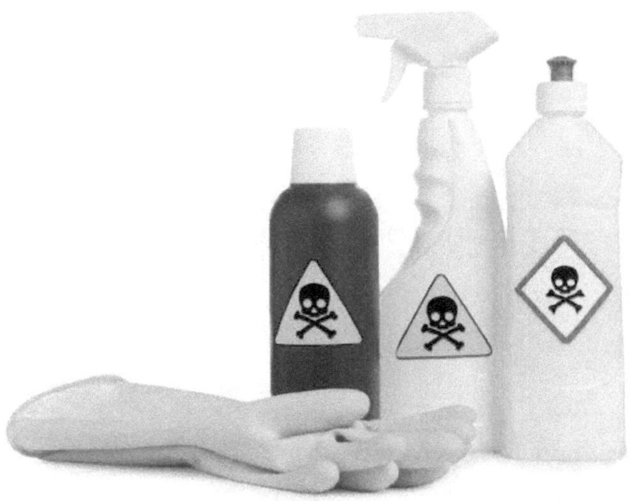

Let's make this real simple by taking some advice from the American Lung Association. Their experts tell us to avoid products with labels that have signal words such as "WARNING," "POISON," or "DANGER." These labels indicate the product within is toxic to humans and animals. So, why in the world would we spray it all over our homes? Remember, when we know better...we do better.

2

Hack #2 Daily Rinsing

This one will be a nice followup to all the inhalants we just discussed. Rewind to my early twenties and my struggle with chronic allergies. I finally got my first piece of natural medicine advice from a doctor to help not just treat, but actually prevent and manage my allergies. It was a nasal saline rinse. Maybe you've heard of this. Rinses come in a variety of forms. My preferred form has been the neti pot for many years.

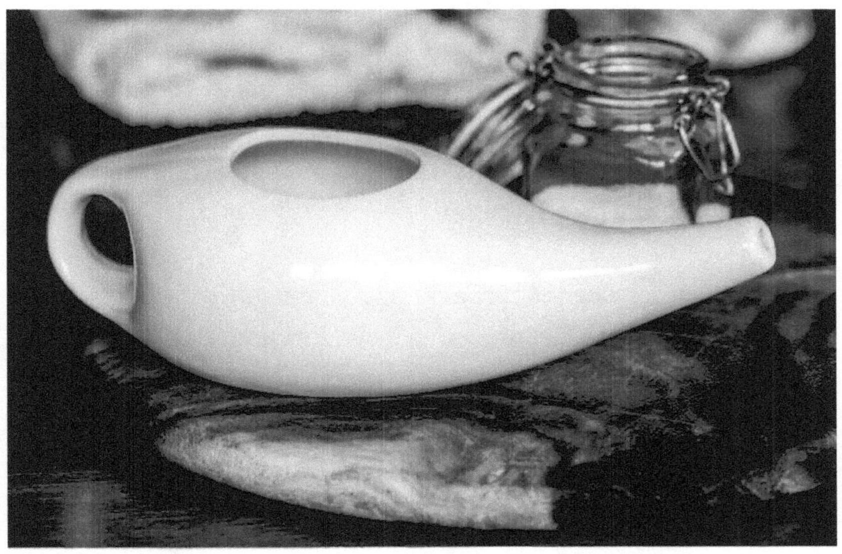

I used to only complete a rinse when I was not feeling well and wanted to rinse out my congested sinuses. Eventually I figured out if I simply rinsed at the end of each day, I could minimize the effects I felt from everyday irritants like dust, dirt, pollen, ragweed, etc. I am reactive to all these things and more.

So, when my kids got their first colds, naturally I was reaching for a rinse to unclog those nasal passages. Of course when they were tiny, I used the snot suckers like many parents use on their small and sensitive nostrils. I'd use a gentle mist of a nasal saline spray to moisten the nostrils and help break up the mucus so I could more easily clear their passages. As they got older, however, I started using a gentle nasal rinse each night to clean out the junk from the day. Because I started with them so early, it's just second nature to them now. Which makes life much easier when they do get a cold and we have to really hit those rinses hard.

Now, they are only 6 and 4 years old as I'm writing this so neither of them use a neti pot like I do. We simply purchased glass nasal spray bottles and nasal saline solution. I keep those filled at home for daily use. Our routine is 3 sprays in each nostril x 3 rounds. If they're sick, we do it until they can breathe better.

Using nasal rinses when you are a chronic allergy sufferer or when you're sick just makes sense, but in case you love data and facts, UCLA Health found that patients with chronic sinus issues who used a daily nasal rinse reported an improvement in symptom severity by more than 60%. So, it sounds like I'm not the only one who thinks this makes good sense.

3

Hack #3 Avoid Artificial Food Colorings (AFCs)

This one continues to be a sticky subject to navigate since most people in the US do not think there is anything wrong with AFCs. Like I used to believe, they too, and maybe you, believe if the food is on the shelf at the grocery store then surely it is safe. After all, the FDA wouldn't allow it to be there if it weren't safe, right? Wrong. The FDA uses the "Generally Recognized as Safe" (GRAS) approach, which considers food additives to be safe until proven otherwise. Proven otherwise by human reactions and/or actual research. Isn't that nice, we have been lab rats all these years and never even knew it. On the other hand, the European Food Safety Authority will research and test new food additives before allowing them to be sold and consumed. Get this, not just for products being consumed by humans but they even test animal feeds.

Okay enough about the lack of food quality regulation, let's talk about all the actual evidence that now exists from all these years of human testing, on 80's babies like me. Honestly, I didn't get serious about avoiding AFCs until I had children. I knew there were negative effects from AFCs on brain function and behavior in children already documented so I was not taking any chances on my littles. But, for myself, I was less concerned because I'm an adult and surely I can handle it. I wasn't worried about me throwing myself on the floor in a full tantrum after I ate a cupcake with pink icing. After doing some additional research for this chapter, my eyes have been opened wide. My mind is slightly blown and I hope I'm about to wake up a few friends with these next few paragraphs.

Did you know there are actually forms of AFCs that can cross the blood-brain barrier? This barrier of cells is present to protect our brains from harmful substances which would disrupt our central nervous system. Even in adults, these artificial dyes can cross our fully developed blood-brain barriers, so it's no surprise they throw our children's developing brains for a major loop. It should not be a surprise that they have a harder time focusing, attending to tasks, and controlling their emotions and behaviors after exposure to AFCs. Of course, we often have a double whammy because many times the AFCs kids are consuming are paired with a big heap of refined sugar, i.e., candy, cookies, junk foods, etc. There's a boatload of research showing how refined sugar negatively impacts brain function, not to mention a pile of other health conditions.

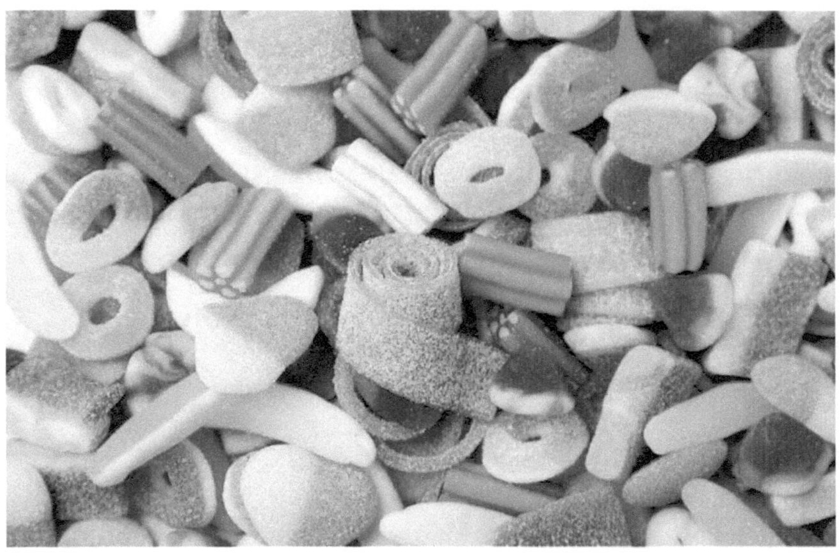

Another fact I learned about consuming AFCs is they have been proven to produce a histamine reaction in some children. This means some children will respond with sneezing, itching, and other allergy-like symptoms after consuming AFCs. After learning this, a huge light bulb went off and made me think back to how I suffered for so long with allergies. During that same time, I was consuming plenty of candy and other junk food that contained AFCs, and of course it's partner in crime, good ole refined sugar. It's no wonder I stayed sick so much. And it's also no wonder I started to stay well, and heal faster when I did get sick, once I started making better food choices. Back in my twenties, I was not thinking that minimizing my consumption of sugary drinks and candy would make my allergies easier to control but in hindsight it is 100% correlated. I'm basically my very own evidence-based research study.

Obviously, a simple way to avoid AFCs is to steer clear of junk foods. A less obvious way is to read labels, all labels, because you will be surprised at how many products have sneaked those nasty little rascals in. They want our food to look pretty and they want us to buy more of it, but with zero regard for the health of their consumers. Sadly, there has been more than enough evidence-based research completed to prove AFCs are unsafe for human consumption, yet they continue to fill our grocery store shelves. We have to look out for ourselves and especially the most vulnerable, our precious little ones.

4

Hack #4 Keeping Gut Health in Check

When I laid the book out, I didn't realize what a perfect segway artificial dyes would be to gut health but it certainly is. By reducing your child's exposure to AFCs, you will likely be reducing their exposure to refined sugars simultaneously. This is great news for your child's gut health!

Did you know our intestines are home to 100 trillion organisms, mainly bacteria? We have both good bacteria and bad bacteria. The good bacteria love foods that are good for us like fruits, vegetables and whole grains, while the bad bacteria love foods that are not good for us like candy, fast food, sugary beverages, and other non-nutritious food items.

The gut is responsible for about 70% of our immune response and our good bacteria are what keep our systems in check. By working daily to create a healthy gut environment for our children, we can keep the bad bacteria under control and keep our children healthier and happier. Gut health not only directly affects physical health but also mental health. Children with a poor good to bad bacteria ratio will often exhibit feelings of anxiety, anger, outbursts, difficulty controlling emotions, irritability and difficulty sleeping.

So, how can we help our kids have a healthy gut environment?

- Limit sugary foods which feed the bad bacteria
- Increase intake of high fiber food like fruits, vegetables, and whole grains
- Add in foods with live, active bacteria such as kefir, yogurt (not the sugary, dyed kind), and fermented foods
- Encourage water intake and avoid sugary beverages
- Minimize consumption of processed/packaged foods and fast food
- Avoid unnecessary antibiotics, and if absolutely necessary then be sure to discuss adding a probiotic supplement with your pediatrician

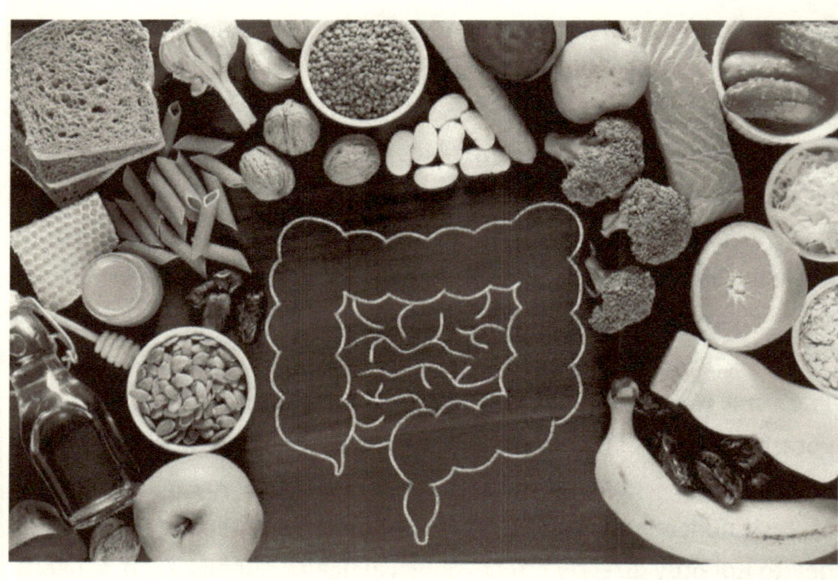

Improving your child's gut health will take time, but it will also require consistency and tenacity on your part. We know all good things take effort and usually some struggles too so hang in there, it will be worth it in the end. Trust me, I've seen first hand what a difference creating a healthy gut environment in your child can make. Our lives have significantly changed as a result of implementing some of these lifestyle changes, and it is 100% worth all the effort.

5

Hack #5 Adding Omega-3s

From infancy, my pediatrician recommended giving my children Omega-3 fatty acids for brain health and development. I greatly respected and trusted my pediatrician and happily complied. As I learned more about the massive benefits of Omega-3s and how much our bodies needed them, I began adding them to my own diet and seeking out foods naturally rich in them.

I am not going to go into immense detail on the scientific facts surrounding Omega-3 fatty acids but I did link several articles in the References section of this book which will give you all the juicy science details if you choose to investigate further. What I do want to give you is what to eat and why it may be beneficial to your child to consume more Omega-3s.

Foods rich in Omega-3s:

- Fish and other seafood (especially cold water, fatty fish like salmon and tuna)
- Nuts and seeds (flax seeds, chia seeds and walnuts for example)
- Plant oils (such as flaxseed, canola or soybean oil)

- Pasture-raised eggs
- Grass-fed meats and dairy products
- Omega-3s in Supplement form may include fish oil, krill oil, cod liver oil

A few benefits your child may experience from the addition of Omega-3s:

- Improved brain growth and brain function
- Improved sleep
- Reduction in symptoms of depression
- Improved control of ADHD symptoms
- Reduction in incidence of allergies
- Support of healthy bone growth

There have been times when we have gotten off track with our daily Omega-3s supplementation and it never takes long to see the difference in my children. When we are consistent with our Omega-3s, we see better attitudes, improved moods, and better ability to focus. Adding Omega-3s is definitely a win for the whole family.

6

Hack #6 Screen Time Limitations

Another controversial topic, and another one I had to agree to disagree on with many friends and family members, including my own husband. We have become a generation in front of screens for better or for worse. I believe we can gain lots of good from computers and such, but if we are not conscientious and self-disciplined we can actually do more harm than good.

First off, screen time offers no benefits to children under the age of 2, but does pose quite a few dangers. This is not just my opinion, it's actually been proven by extremely intelligent scientists who have studied brain activity in young children for many years. Patricia Kuhl is one of the world's leading brain scientists. She studies brain activity in over 4,000 babies a year. From her studies, Patricia has concluded that children under age 1 are unable to learn from a machine. No matter how captivating the videos were, the babies studied were not able to learn new information, based on their brain scans. However, the same babies being taught the same content by a live person demonstrated genius level learning, based on their brain scans.

I'm not the best at rule following, so the opinions of large organizations don't always matter to me but I will still note that the World Health Organization does not recommend screen time for children under age 2, and the American Academy of Pediatrics does not recommend screen time until at least 18 months. In case you don't want to take my word for it, these organizations offer some great advice in this area also.

Now, don't get me wrong, I do believe there are many awesome benefits to technology, especially as a mom who is homeschooling her two kids. There are some great learning activities and educational content within apps and channels that we are grateful to be able to access and learn from. Even with screen time for learning though, I have to be careful they don't stay on too long as someone will always walk away irritable, grumpy and itching to get in trouble. My 4 year old is more sensitive than my 6 year old so his online learning sessions are always shorter than his older sister's sessions. Regardless, we avoid more than 30 minutes consecutively.

Later in the day, if they have demonstrated appropriate and respectful behavior, they will have the opportunity to watch a short show for pure entertainment pleasure. Usually they each get to select 20 minutes of content. If I get distracted and let them go over, I almost always pay the price so I try to set timers and stay on top of it.

In case you are not yet a believer as to why too much screen time can be harmful to our children, I'll list some of the proven side effects which have been well documented by many scientists and struggling parents alike.

Excessive Screen Time Side Effects:

- Difficulty focusing
- Decreased attention to tasks
- Decreased executive function skills (impulse control, self-monitoring, organization, initiation, and more)
- Impaired academic performance
- Reduced frequency and quality of interactions with other children and family
- Impaired social and emotional development
- Increased likelihood of obesity
- Difficulty sleeping
- Increased risk of mental health conditions, including depression and anxiety

We don't need to totally avoid screen time but certainly as parents we need to set healthy boundaries for our children. We cannot expect the children to know how to monitor and regulate themselves in this area. I realize it will be hard to break current habits and start fresh, but it can be done and it will be worth it. One day, like when they are grown and starting to enforce these same guidelines in their own homes, they will thank you.

7

Hack #7 Outdoor Time

My children are so much happier when they are outdoors. It's simply a fact. When they are driving me bonkers in the house, the answer is almost always, "Go outside and play!" Sometimes they give me grief but once they are out the door, it's game on. The adventure begins. Their imaginations engage. They are happy. They are actually getting along and playing without trying to kill each other. It's just so awesome!

Pediatricians recommend school age children spend about 3 hours outside each day. With the demands of most family's busy schedules, this is likely easier said than done. So, what are some benefits of your child getting the recommended amount of outdoor play time? **Let's list a few:**

- Improved physical health of child, combating obesity and other weight-related health concerns
- Improved mental and emotional health of child
- Improved social skills as they play and interact with other children
- Less screen time, which as you've already read will have many

benefits
- Improved sleep habits
- Improved mood
- Stronger immune system as they breathe in fresh air, get Vitamin D from the sun, and are exposed to microorganisms in the soil.

With all these wonderful benefits, hopefully you are now more motivated to get those kiddos outdoors every day. Let them play and get dirty. Encourage their imaginations to run wild. I like to send mine out while I am fixing dinner and then again as I'm cleaning up the mess from dinner. Gives me a mental break and they get to squeeze out the last benefits of the outdoors for the day.

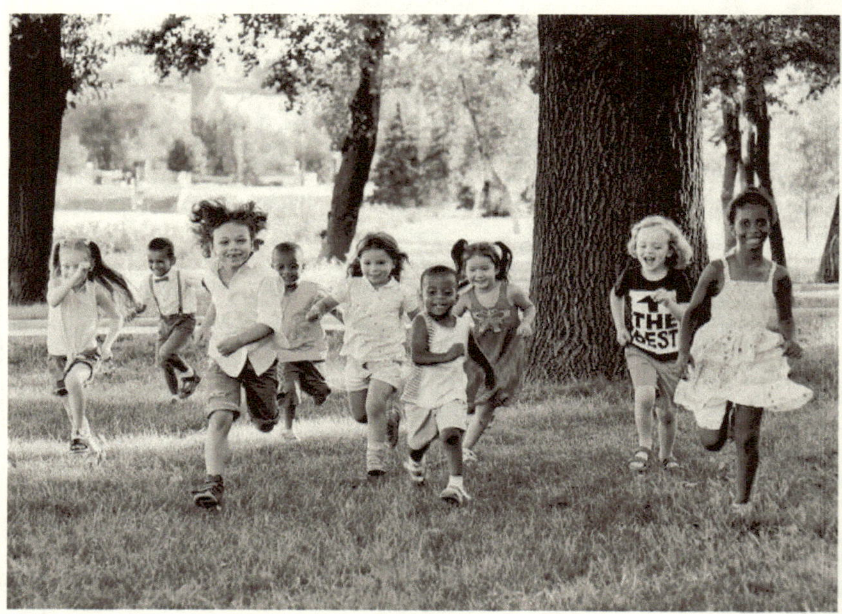

Here some fun ideas to get your family outdoors more:

- Scavenger Hunt- There are lots of free downloads you can print out or just make up your own.
- Plant something together- It can be in a small pot, a raised bed, or the ground. They will just have so much fun digging in the dirt.
- Outdoor games like "Simon says", "Mother May I?", and "Red Light Green Light"
- Make an Obstacle Course in the yard
- Visit a local playground or park
- Make houses or terrariums for worms or bugs you find in the yard using mason jars. They are fun to make and watch the critters before releasing them.
- Create leaf rubbings- Find leaves, place them under a piece of paper, then color the paper to create a leaf impression.
- Take a walk or do a workout together
- Have a picnic, or simply take dinner out to the porch or patio

Hopefully that list got your ideas flowing and will encourage you to get outdoors with your children more often.

8

Hack #8 Support from Nature

I'm going to preface this chapter by stating I am not a doctor, nor am I attempting to be with anything I have shared, or am about to share, in this book. I am simply a person who has lived out a lifestyle change for almost 2 decades now, and seen first hand the benefits of utilizing these practices in my own life and in the lives of my children.

I fully believe we have very smart bodies, because we have an all-knowing Creator. Our bodies know how to heal themselves from everyday illnesses and injuries. I also believe there is a natural remedy for everything that ails us somewhere on this earth. It's just a matter of finding out the right blend, dosage, quantity, etc.

Traditional medicine, the use of knowledge, skills, and practices to prevent and treat illnesses, is documented back at least 3000 years. This line of medicine uses herbal remedies, derived from nature, to aid the body in natural healing. Whereas, conventional medicine started a little over 100 years ago. Instead of using nature to promote healing, conventional medicine uses laboratories to create chemical, synthetic

24

medications. I don't know about you, but I vote for remedies derived from nature and backed by centuries of evidence, over 100 years of lab rats.

I've already talked about many of our practices for prevention of illness, but let's talk about what we do when the kids do get sick. First of all, we don't rush them to med express or call their doctor because they have a snotty nose, sore throat, fever, achy stomach, etc. We do encourage extra rest, hydration and the use of herbal remedies.

I have a cabinet full of tinctures to treat most common illnesses. Tinctures are concentrated herbal extracts that are formed by soaking parts of plants for a period of time in alcohol or vinegar. This process extracts the plant's most powerful benefits, which we then use to aid our bodies in the natural healing process.

When sickness strikes the homefront, we also whip up a brew of homemade elderberry syrup. The one who is sick gets numerous doses a day and the rest of us take at least one dose for prevention, and more if we start to feel symptoms as well. I'm adding my preferred recipe below in case you want to try it out. It's really simple, it just takes a little time and effort. It can be a messy process but worth it in the end. Or just buy some homemade from a local source you trust.

Elderberry Syrup:

- 3 ½ C water
- ⅔ C dried organic elderberries
- 2 TBSP ginger grated
- 2 organic cinnamon sticks (or 1 tsp ground cinnamon)
- 1 tsp whole organic cloves (or ½ tsp ground cloves)

- 1 C raw, local honey

Instructions:

1. Add all ingredients EXCEPT honey to a large pot.
2. Cover with lid, then bring to boil.
3. Remove lid and reduce to simmer for approx. 30 minutes or until liquid is reduced by half.
4. Remove from heat and allow to cool to lukewarm.
5. Remove the cinnamon sticks and whole cloves. Smash the berries to get the juices out while still in the pot.
6. Pour through a mesh strainer or cheesecloth over a bowl or jar. I prefer bowl.
7. Ensuring the liquid is no longer hot, add the Honey and stir well.
8. Pour into a jar and enjoy
9. Standard dosages are ½ to 1 tsp for kids and ½ to 1 TBSP for adults. Once a day for prevention and every 2-3 hours if fighting an illness.

Another remedy we utilize, and strongly believe in, is what I fondly call "immunity tea". I created this blend when I was pregnant with my first child and had gotten a cold. I refused to take any over the counter medications but I had quite the raging cold going on. This blend was so soothing and helped me heal quickly and without conventional medicine. Whenever we feel a sniffle starting, we hit it with a few cups of this tea blend.

<u>Immunity Tea Blend:</u>

- 1 TBSP dried, organic Echinacea
- 1 TBSP dried, organic Burdock Root

- 1 TBSP dried, organic Marshmallow Root
- 1 TBSP dried, organic Rosehips

Instructions:

1. You will need a Loose Leaf Tea Infuser and a pot to make this. You do not need a designated tea pot but I love mine.
2. Boil water.
3. Add infuser/s to the pot.
4. Pour boiling water over the infusers.
5. Wait 20 minutes.
6. Enjoy the tea.
7. We usually add raw, local honey for pleasure, but also to soothe sore throats and coughs.

Speaking of coughs, a lifesaver for us has been using Colloidal Silver in a pediatric nebulizer. We bought one for about $35.00 at a local pharmacy a few years ago. It is adorable, it looks like a puppy dog so it's super non-threatening to the kids. We use a pediatric face mask to increase the likelihood of them actually inhaling the soothing vapors. We fill the medicine cup with a dropper full, or two, of Colloidal Silver and let it run while we read books. When the steam stops coming, we take it off. This simple strategy has saved us from so many sleepless nights due to coughing. It also has proven to help my kids kick the coughs much more quickly. It does take extra time and effort, but it is 100% worth it.

The last intervention I'll mention is the use of bentonite clay. I recommend the "Redmond" brand. This clay can be used for so many things so research it more, but I'll note a few that we use it for. Bee stings, bug bites, scratches, burns, and poison ivy to name a few. Simply add some clay (it's in a powder form) to a small bowl. Add enough water to make a paste. Apply to whatever area is troubling you.

28

A few years ago, I cut my finger very deep. Maybe I could have used a few stitches. Instead I gobbed a clay paste onto the finger, wrapped it, and repeated this process for several days. About a week later, my finger was healed and I didn't even have a scar to show for it. Keep it in stock and take it with you when you travel. You'll be glad you did!

9

Conclusion

This has really been fun writing all this down. I'm not sure how many people will actually read it but if you are reading this, then I sure hope you gleaned a thing or two from it that will bless your family.

I hope you will be encouraged to spend more time outdoors with your children. I hope you will start reading labels and digging deeper into why AFCs and processed foods are so damaging to the health of our children. I hope you will learn to trust nature to help heal your children's bodies naturally. I hope you will have fun teaching your children about all that you are learning and why it's so important to begin making these changes as a family.

Thank you for taking the time to read this and invest in the health and happiness of your children. All we want as parents is to have healthy, happy kids, and these "hacks" will be a great start.

Disclaimer: As I already stated, I am not a doctor. Please if you or your children are being treated by a doctor for any reason or you take any medications, please confirm with your healthcare provider before starting any new supplements or herbal remedies to prevent any unwanted interactions.

10

Author's Favs

ere is a list of a few of my preferred vendors, websites, and/or which you may find helpful as you begin your journey towards a healthier, happier home:

1. *Melaleuca, The Wellness Company:* I get many of our supplements, all of our cleaning and laundry supplies, and some of our personal care items from here. USA made. I am a part of their affiliate program so if you use this link, I will get financial credit for referring you there. http://melaleuca.com/ashleylumpkins
2. *Earthley:* I get all of our tinctures and some of our personal care items from here. USA made. I am a part of their affiliate program so if you use this link, I will get financial credit for referring you there. https://www.earthley.com/ref/alumpkins/
3. *YumEarth:* Organic Candy that is allergy friendly, free from AFCs, and really yummy. A great alternative treat for the kids. I take these to birthday parties, trade out at Halloween, etc so they aren't eating the other toxic candies but are still getting some special treats.
4. *Alkolol:* This is nasal rinse sold on Amazon. I fill their nasal spray bottles ¾ full with saline solution then top them off with this

product.

5. *Frontier Co-op:* I buy many of my dried herbs for making tea from this co-op. You can find at several online stores but I usually get mine from Amazon.

6. *Azure Standard:* Look this one up for sure. Excellent resource for all things organic and natural. Bulk orders. Great prices. I shop here for lots of food needs.

11

Resources

CT Dept of Energy and Environmental Protection. (2018, August). *Household alternatives for reducing toxic products in your home.* CT.gov - Connecticut's Official State Website. Retrieved October 6, 2024, from https://portal.ct.gov/deep/p2/individual/household-alt ernatives-for-reducing-toxic-products-in-your-home

American Lung Association. (2024, July 29). *Cleaning supplies and household chemicals.* lung.org. Retrieved October 6, 2024, from https://w ww.lung.org/clean-air/indoor-air/indoor-air-pollutants/cleaning-su pplies-household-chem

Melaleuca The Wellness Company. (2024). *Toxic Chemical in National Brand Cleaners.* Melaleuca. Retrieved October 6, 2024, from https://ww w.melaleuca.com/productstore/lung-study

Melaleuca The Wellness Company. (2024a). *The Power of Nature.* Melaleuca. Retrieved October 6, 2024, from https://www.melaleuca. com/our-story/ingredients-philosophy

UCLA Health. (2022, May 2). *Risks and rewards of nasal rinses: What you need to know.* Retrieved October 6, 2024, from https://www.uclahea lth.org/news/article/risks-and-rewards-of-nasal-rinses-what-you- need-to-know

D. Miller, M. et al. (2022). Potential impacts of synthetic food dyes on activity and attention in children: a review of the human and animal evidence. *Environmental Health.* https://www.ncbi.nlm.nih.gov/pmc/articles/PMC9052604/

Organic Soda Pops. (2024, August 10). *5 American food ingredients that are banned in Europe and other parts of the world.* Retrieved October 6, 2024, from https://organicsodapops.com/blogs/news/5-american-food-ingredients-that-are-banned-in-europe-and-other-parts-of-the-world?_pos=1&_sid=88bad7d27&_ss=r

Kashyap, R. et al. (2016). A Review of the Association of Blue Food Coloring With Attention Deficit Hyperactivity Disorder Symptoms in Children. *Cureus*, PMID: 36262950. https://www.ncbi.nlm.nih.gov/pmc/articles/PMC9573786/#:~:text

Stanford Medicine. (2024). *5 ways to boost your child's gut health.* Stanford Medicine Children's Health. Retrieved October 6, 2024, from https://www.stanfordchildrens.org/en/topic/default?id=5-ways-to-boost-your-childs-gut-health-197-29161

Subramani, A. (2023, September 1). *The importance of good gut health in children.* Only About Children. Retrieved October 6, 2024, from https://www.oac.edu.au/news-views/the-importance-of-good-gut-health-in-children/

5 tips for building better gut health in kids. (2022, September 28). Children's Hospital of Richmond at VCU. Retrieved October 6, 2024, from https://www.chrichmond.org/blog/5-tips-for-building-better-gut-health-in-kids

Bartholomew, R. (2022, August 29). *Top 10 reasons to give your kids omega-3 | Nutri Advanced.* Nutri Advanced. Retrieved October 6, 2024, from https://www.nutriadvanced.co.uk/news/top-10-reasons-to-give-your-kids-omega-3/

Office of Dietary Supplements. (2022, July 18). *Omega-3 fatty acids.* NIH National Institutes of Health. Retrieved October 7, 2024, from https://ods.od.nih.gov/factsheets/Omega3FattyAcids-Consumer/

Nelson, C. (n.d.). *Babies need humans, not screens.* Unicef. Retrieved October 7, 2024, from https://www.unicef.org/parenting/child-develo pment/babies-screen-time#:~:text=

Kumar Muppalla, S. (2023). Effects of Excessive Screen Time on Child Development: An Updated Review and Strategies for Management. *Cureus.* https://www.ncbi.nlm.nih.gov/pmc/articles/PMC10353947/

Fliesler, N. (2023, February 2). *Screen time caution for babies – Boston Children's Answers.* Boston Children's Answers. Retrieved October 7, 2024, from https://answers.childrenshospital.org/screen-time-infant s/

Johnson, A. (2022, March 9). *Screen time recommendations by age.* All About Vision. Retrieved October 7, 2024, from https://www.allaboutvisi on.com/conditions/refractive-errors/screen-time-by-age/#:~:text=

K. Lockwood, K. (2024, March 13). *The Benefits of Outdoor Play: Why it Matters.* Children's Hospital of Philadelphia. Retrieved October 7, 2024, from https://www.chop.edu/news/health-tip/benefits-outdoor-play-why-it-matters#:~:text=

Ayuob, M. (2024, May 29). *5 ways slimming screen time is good for your health.* Mayo Clinic. Retrieved October 7, 2024, from https://www.ma yoclinichealthsystem.org/hometown-health/featured-topic/5-ways-slimming-screen-time-is-good-for-your-health#:~:text=

Garcia-Navarro, L. (2017, July 16). "Dirt is Good": Why kids need exposure to germs. *NPR.* https://www.npr.org/sections/health-shots/ 2017/07/16/537075018/dirt-is-good-why-kids-need-exposure-to-g erms

Administrator. (2020, April 1). *Sunbathing can boost your body's immune system.* Universitas Gadjah Mada. Retrieved October 7, 2024, from https://ugm.ac.id/en/news/19216-sunbathing-can-boost-your-body-s-immune-system/#:~:text=

Wachtel-Galor, S., & Benzie, I. F. F. (2011). *Herbal Medicine.* Herbal

Medicine - NCBI Bookshelf. Retrieved October 7, 2024, from https://www.ncbi.nlm.nih.gov/books/NBK92773/

[Historical sketch of modern pharmaceutical science and technology (Part 3). From the second half of the 19th century to World War II]. (1995). PubMed. Retrieved October 7, 2024, from https://pubmed.ncbi.nlm.nih.gov/11613518/#:~:text=

Cirino, E. (2023, July 13). *What you need to know about herbal tinctures.* Healthline. Retrieved October 7, 2024, from https://www.healthline.com/health/what-is-a-tincture